Copyright © 2020 by J

All rights reserved. No part of this publication may be reproduced, distributed, or transmitted in any form or by any means, including photocopying, recording, or other electronic or mechanical methods, without the prior written permission of the publisher, except in the case of brief quotations embodied in critical reviews and certain other noncommercial uses permitted by copyright law

Contents

A Beginner's Guide to the Low-FODMAP Diet 5

What Are FODMAPs? 5

Benefits of a Low-FODMAP Diet 7

Increased Quality of Life 9

Who Should Follow a Low-FODMAP Diet 10

How to Follow a Low-FODMAP Diet 12

A Low-FODMAP Diet Can Be Flavorful 19

Can Vegetarians Follow a Low-FODMAP Diet? 21

A Sample Low-FODMAP Shopping List 22

What If Your Symptoms Don't Improve? 24

Pumpkin Layer Cake 28

LOW FODMAP PUMPKIN GINGERBREAD STREUSEL COFFEE CAKE 35

LEMONY LOW FODMAP CARBONARA 41

MATZO BALL SOUP 46

FODMAP CUCUMBER GAZPACHO 51

LOW FODMAP SPICY SMOKY PUMPKIN SOUP 54

LOW FODMAP VEGETABLE, PASTA & BEAN SOUP 59

LOW FODMAP BOUILLABAISSE 64

LOW FODMAP GAZPACHO 72

LOW FODMAP VEGETABLE BROTH 77

LOW FODMAP CLAM CHOWDER 84

LOW FODMAP OYSTER MUSHROOM GRAVY 92

LOW FODMAP SPOOKY GRAVEYARD 7-LAYER DIP 96

LOW FODMAP SWEET & SPICY DRY RUB 101

LOW FODMAP PINEAPPLE SALSA 104

LOW FODMAP RED WINE VINAIGRETTE 107

LOW FODMAP MINT SALSA VERDE 110

LOW FODMAP MISO COD RAMEN 113

A Beginner's Guide to the Low-FODMAP Diet

Food is a common trigger of digestive symptoms. Interestingly, restricting certain foods can dramatically improve these symptoms in sensitive people.

In particular, a diet low in fermentable carbs known as FODMAPS is clinically recommended for the management of irritable bowel syndrome (IBS).

This book explains what a low-FODMAP diet is, how it works and who should try it.

What Are FODMAPs?

FODMAP stands for fermentable oligo-, di-, mono-saccharides and polyols (1Trusted Source).

These are the scientific terms used to classify groups of carbs that are notorious for triggering digestive symptoms like bloating, gas and stomach pain.

FODMAPs are found in a wide range of foods in varying amounts. Some foods contain just one type, while others contain several.

The main dietary sources of the four groups of FODMAPs include:

• Oligosaccharides: Wheat, rye, legumes and various fruits and vegetables, such as garlic and onions.

• Disaccharides: Milk, yogurt and soft cheese. Lactose is the main carb.

• Monosaccharides: Various fruit including figs and mangoes, and sweeteners such as honey and agave nectar. Fructose is the main carb.

- Polyols: Certain fruits and vegetables including blackberries and lychee, as well as some low-calorie sweeteners like those in sugar-free gum.

SUMMARY:

FODMAPs are a group of fermentable carbs that aggravate gut symptoms in sensitive people. They're found in a wide range of foods.

Benefits of a Low-FODMAP Diet

A low-FODMAP diet restricts high-FODMAP foods.

The benefits of a low-FODMAP diet have been tested in thousands of people with IBS across more than 30 studies (2Trusted Source).

Reduced Digestive Symptoms

IBS digestive symptoms can vary widely, including stomach pain, bloating, reflux, flatulence and bowel urgency.

Stomach pain is a hallmark of the condition, and bloating has been found to affect more than 80% of people with IBS.

Needless to say, these symptoms can be debilitating. One large study even reported that people with IBS said they would give up an average of 25% of their remaining lives to be symptom-free (5Trusted Source).

Fortunately, both stomach pain and bloating have been shown to significantly decrease with a low-FODMAP diet.

Evidence from four high-quality studies concluded that if you follow a low-FODMAP diet, your odds of improving stomach pain and bloating are 81% and 75% greater, respectively (2Trusted Source).

Several other studies have suggested the diet can help manage flatulence, diarrhea and constipation.

Increased Quality of Life

People with IBS often report a reduced quality of life, and severe digestive symptoms have been associated with this.

Luckily, several studies have found the low-FODMAP diet improves overall quality of life (2Trusted Source).

There is also some evidence showing that a low-FODMAP diet may increase energy levels in people with IBS, but placebo-controlled studies are needed to support this finding (6Trusted Source).

SUMMARY:

There is convincing evidence for the benefits of a low-FODMAP diet. The diet appears to improve digestive symptoms in approximately 70% of adults with IBS.

Who Should Follow a Low-FODMAP Diet

A low-FODMAP diet is not for everyone. Unless you have been diagnosed with IBS, research suggests the diet could do more harm than good.

This is because most FODMAPs are prebiotics, meaning they support the growth of good gut bacteria (10Trusted Source).

Also, most of the research has been in adults. Therefore, there is limited support for the diet in children with IBS.

If you have IBS, consider this diet if you:

- Have ongoing gut symptoms.

- Haven't responded to stress management strategies.

- Haven't responded to first-line dietary advice, including restricting alcohol, caffeine, spicy food and other common trigger foods (11)Trusted Source.

That said, there is some speculation that the diet may benefit other conditions, including diverticulitis and exercise-induced digestive issues. More research is underway.

It is important to be aware that the diet is an involved process. For this reason, it's not recommended to try it for the first time while traveling or during a busy or stressful period.

SUMMARY:A low-FODMAP diet is recommended for adults with IBS. The evidence for its use in other conditions is limited and may do more harm than good.

How to Follow a Low-FODMAP Diet

A low-FODMAP diet is more complex than you may think and involves three stages.

Stage 1: Restriction

This stage involves strict avoidance of all high-FODMAP foods.

People who follow this diet often think they should avoid all FODMAPs long-term, but this stage should only last about 3–8 weeks. This is because it's important to include FODMAPs in the diet for gut health.

Some people notice an improvement in symptoms in the first week, while others take the full eight weeks. Once you have adequate relief of your digestive symptoms, you can progress to the second stage.

If by eight weeks your gut symptoms have not resolved, refer to the What If Your Symptoms Don't Improve? chapter below.

Stage 2: Reintroduction

This stage involves systematically reintroducing high-FODMAP foods.

The purpose of this is twofold:

1. To identify which types of FODMAPs you tolerate. Few people are sensitive to all of them.

2. To establish the amount of FODMAPs you can tolerate. This is known as your "threshold level."

In this step, you test specific foods one by one for three days each (1Trusted Source).

It is recommended that you undertake this step with a trained dietitian who can guide you through the appropriate foods. Alternatively, this app can help you identify which foods to reintroduce.

It is worth noting that you need to continue a low-FODMAP diet throughout this stage. This means even if you can tolerate a certain high-FODMAP food, you must continue to restrict it until stage 3.

It is also important to remember that, unlike people with most food allergies, people with IBS can tolerate small amounts of FODMAPs.

Lastly, although digestive symptoms can be debilitating, they will not cause long-term damage to your body.

Stage 3: Personalization

This stage is also known as the "modified low-FODMAP diet." In other words, you still restrict some FODMAPs. However, the amount and type are tailored to your personal tolerance, identified in stage 2.

It is important to progress to this final stage in order to increase diet variety and flexibility. These qualities are linked with improved long-term compliance, quality of life and gut health (14Trusted Source).

You can find a video explaining this three-stage process here.

SUMMARY:

Many people are surprised to find that the low-FODMAP diet is a three-stage process. Each stage is equally important in achieving long-term symptom relief and overall health and well-being.

Three Things to Do Before You Get Started

There are three things you should do before embarking on the diet.

1. Make Sure You Actually Have IBS

Digestive symptoms can occur in many conditions, some harmless and others more serious.

Unfortunately, there is no positive diagnostic test to confirm you have IBS. For this reason, it is recommended you see a doctor to rule out more serious conditions first, such as celiac disease, inflammatory bowel disease and colon cancer (15Trusted Source).

Once these are ruled out, your doctor can confirm you have IBS using the official IBS diagnostic criteria — you must fulfill all three to be diagnosed with IBS (4Trusted Source):

- Recurrent stomach pain: On average, at least one day per week in the last three months.

- Stool symptoms: These should match two or more of the following: related to defecation, associated with a change in frequency of stool or associated with a change in the appearance of stool.

- Persistent symptoms: Criteria fulfilled for the last three months with symptom onset at least six months before diagnosis.

2. Try First-Line Diet Strategies

The low-FODMAP diet is a time- and resource-intensive process.

This is why in clinical practice it is considered second-line dietary advice and is only used in a subset of people with IBS who don't respond to first-line strategies.

More information about first-line dietary advice can be found here.

3. Plan Ahead

The diet can be difficult to follow if you are not prepared. Here are some tips:

• Find out what to buy: Ensure you have access to credible low-FODMAP food lists. See below for a list of where to find these.

• Get rid of high-FODMAP foods: Clear your fridge and pantry of these foods.

• Make a shopping list: Create a low-FODMAP shopping list before heading to the grocery store, so you know which foods to purchase or avoid.

- Read menus in advance: Familiarize yourself with low-FODMAP menu options so you'll be prepared when dining out.

SUMMARY:

Before you embark on the low-FODMAP diet, there are several things you need to do. These simple steps will help increase your chances of successfully managing your digestive symptoms.

A Low-FODMAP Diet Can Be Flavorful

Garlic and onion are both very high in FODMAPs. This has led to the common misconception that a low-FODMAP diet lacks flavor.

While many recipes do use onion and garlic for flavor, there are many low-FODMAP herbs, spices and savory flavorings that can be substituted instead.

It is also worth highlighting that you can still get the flavor from garlic using strained garlic-infused oil, which is low in FODMAPs.

This is because the FODMAPs in garlic are not fat-soluble, meaning the garlic flavor is transferred to the oil, but the FODMAPs aren't.

Other low-FODMAP suggestions: Chives, chili, fenugreek, ginger, lemongrass, mustard seeds, pepper, saffron and turmeric .

SUMMARY:

Several popular flavors are high in FODMAPs, but there are many low-FODMAP herbs and spices that can be used to make flavorsome meals.

Can Vegetarians Follow a Low-FODMAP Diet?

A well-balanced vegetarian diet can be low in FODMAPs. Nonetheless, following a low-FODMAP diet if you are a vegetarian can be more challenging.

This is because high-FODMAP legumes are staple protein foods in vegetarian diets.

That said, you can include small portions of canned and rinsed legumes in a low-FODMAP diet. Serving sizes are typically about 1/4 cup (64 grams).

There are also many low-FODMAP, protein-rich options for vegetarians, including tempeh, tofu, eggs, Quorn (a meat substitute) and most nuts and seeds (19Trusted Source).

SUMMARY:

There are many protein-rich vegetarian options suitable for a low-FODMAP diet. Therefore, there is no reason why a vegetarian with IBS cannot follow a well-balanced low-FODMAP diet.

A Sample Low-FODMAP Shopping List

Many foods are naturally low in FODMAPs.

Here is a simple shopping list to get you started.

- Protein: Beef, chicken, eggs, fish, lamb, pork, prawns and tofu

- Whole grains: Brown rice, buckwheat, maize, millet, oats and quinoa

- Fruit: Bananas, blueberries, kiwi, limes, mandarins, oranges, papaya, pineapple, rhubarb and strawberries

- Vegetables: Bean sprouts, bell peppers, carrots, choy sum, eggplant, kale, tomatoes, spinach and zucchini
- Nuts: Almonds (no more than 10 per sitting), macadamia nuts, peanuts, pecans, pine nuts and walnuts
- Seeds: Linseeds, pumpkin, sesame and sunflower
- Dairy: Cheddar cheese, lactose-free milk and Parmesan cheese
- Oils: Coconut oil and olive oil
- Beverages: Black tea, coffee, green tea, peppermint tea, water and white tea
- Condiments: Basil, chili, ginger, mustard, pepper, salt, white rice vinegar and wasabi powder

Additionally, it's important to check the ingredients list on packaged foods for added FODMAPs.

Food companies may add FODMAPs to their foods for many reasons, including as prebiotics, as a fat substitute or as a lower-calorie substitute for sugar.

SUMMARY:

Many foods are naturally low in FODMAPs. That said, many processed foods have added FODMAPs and should be limited.

What If Your Symptoms Don't Improve?

The low-FODMAP diet does not work for everyone with IBS. Around 30% of people don't respond to the diet (20Trusted Source).

Fortunately, there are other non-diet-based therapies that may help. Talk to your doctor about alternative options.

That said, before you give up on the low-FODMAP diet, you should:

1. Check and Recheck Ingredient Lists

Prepackaged foods often contain hidden sources of FODMAPs.

Common culprits include onion, garlic, sorbitol and xylitol, which can trigger symptoms even in small amounts.

2. Consider the Accuracy of Your FODMAP Information

There are many low-FODMAP food lists available online.

However, there are only two universities that provide comprehensive, validated FODMAP food lists and apps — King's College London and Monash University.

3. Think About Other Life Stressors

Diet is not the only thing that can aggravate IBS symptoms. Stress is another major contributor (21Trusted Source).

In fact, no matter how effective your diet, if you are under severe stress, your symptoms are likely to persist.

SUMMARY:The low-FODMAP diet does not work for everyone. However, there are common mistakes worth checking before you try other therapies.

The Bottom Line

The low-FODMAP diet can dramatically improve digestive symptoms, including those in people with IBS.

However, not everyone with IBS responds to the diet. What's more, the diet involves a three-stage process that can take up to six months.

And unless you need it, the diet may do more harm than good, since FODMAPs are prebiotics that support the growth of beneficial bacteria in your gut.

Nonetheless, this diet could be truly life-changing for those struggling with IBS.

Pumpkin Layer Cake

Our Low FODMAP Pumpkin Layer Cake is easy to make, and yields dramatic results. Make sure to read the recipe through before starting. You might need to order the black cocoa ahead of time.

Makes: 12 Servings

Prep Time: 20 minutes

Cook Time: 35 minutes

Total Time: 55 minutes

INGREDIENTS:

Pumpkin Layer Cake:

- 2 cups (290 g) low FODMAP gluten-free all-purpose flour, such as Bob's Red Mill 1 to 1 Gluten Free Baking Flour

- 2 teaspoons baking powder; use gluten-free if following a gluten-free diet
- 1 teaspoon baking soda
- ¾ teaspoon salt
- 1, 15- ounce (425 g) can of pure pumpkin purée, such as Libby's
- 3/4 cup (180 ml) vegetable oil such as canola, rice bran or sunflower
- ¾ cup (149 g) sugar
- 1/2 cup (107 g) firmly packed light brown sugar
- 4 large eggs, at room temperature
- 1 1/2 teaspoon cinnamon
- 1 1/4 teaspoons ground ginger
- 1 teaspoon vanilla extract

Black Cocoa Frosting:

- ½ cup (113 g) unsalted butter, melted

- 2/3 cup (62 g) sifted black cocoa

- 3 cups (270 g) sifted confectioners' sugar

- 3 to 6 tablespoons lactose-free whole milk

- 1 teaspoon vanilla extract

PREPARATION:

1. Make the Cake: Position rack in center of oven. Preheat oven to 350°F (180°C). Coat the inside of a three, 6-inch (15 cbaking pans with nonstick spray, line with parchment paper, then spritz the paper, too. Set aside.

2. In a large bowl, whisk together the flour, baking powder, baking soda and salt to aerate and combine. Make a well in the center of the dry mixture and set aside.

3. In a separate bowl, whisk together the oil, pumpkin, sugar, brown sugar, eggs, cinnamon, ground ginger and vanilla until well blended. Scrape this pumpkin mixture over the dry and whisk everything together very well. Scrape into prepared pans, dividing evenly, leveling the top. Batter will be thick.

4. Bake for about 30 to 40 minutes or until a toothpick inserted in the center tests clean. Cool pans on rack for about 5 minutes or until just warm. Unmold onto rack, remove parchment and cool completely.

5. Make the Frosting: Pour the melted butter into a mixing bowl and beat in the cocoa on medium speed

using an electric mixer until combined. Slowly beat in confectioners' sugar alternately with 3 tablespoons of milk. Keep beating until super silky smooth, scraping down bowl as needed. Beat in vanilla and beat in additional milk if needed to make a smooth, spreadable frosting.

6. Assembly: Trim cake layers if needed to create level layers. Place one cake layer, top side up, on display plate and frost the top. Place second cake layer, top side up down top of frosting and frost that layer's top as well. Place final layer bottom side up on top of your stacked layers and frost the top and sides either generously with the icing for a smooth look, or use less icing for a schmeared-on look allowing the orange cake to show through. An icing spatula will help make the process easy

in either case. Cake is ready to serve or may be stored under a cake dome at room temperature for up to 2 days.

Tips

• A cake decorating turntable and a few different icing spatulas of various shapes and sizes will make decorating any cake easier and help you achieve professional looking results. They are not necessary, but if you like to bake and decorate cakes, I highly suggest looking into these tools.

• I sourced many of the decorations that you see in the images at the dollar store! Always a great source for holiday décor.

Course: Dessert

Cuisine: American

NUTRITION

Calories: 413kcal | Carbohydrates: 49g | Protein: 5g | Fat: 23g | Saturated Fat: 1g | Sodium: 315mg | Fiber: 2g | Sugar: 24g | Calcium: 3mg | Iron: 1mg

LOW FODMAP PUMPKIN GINGERBREAD STREUSEL COFFEE CAKE

This might be the PERFECT fall coffee cake - for bake sales, guests, host gifts...we like discovering excuses to make it!

Makes: 14 Servings

Prep Time: 10 minutes

Cook Time: 50 minutes

Total Time: 1 hour

INGREDIENTS:

Brown Sugar Spiced Streusel:

- ¼ cup (54 g) firmly packed light brown sugar
- ¼ cup (50 g) sugar

- ¼ cup (36 g) low FODMAP gluten-free all-purpose flour, such as Bob's Red Mill 1 to 1 Gluten Free Baking Flour

- 3 tablespoons unsalted butter, softened

- 1 ½ teaspoons cinnamon

- ½ teaspoon ground ginger

- 1/8 teaspoon ground cloves

- 1/8 teaspoon freshly grated nutmeg

- ¾ cup (75 g) pecan halves, chopped

Pumpkin Gingerbread Coffee Cake:

- 1 ¾ cups (254 g) plus 2 tablespoons low FODMAP gluten-free all-purpose flour, such as Bob's Red Mill 1 to 1 Gluten Free Baking Flour

- 2 teaspoons baking powder; use gluten-free if following a gluten-free diet

- ½ teaspoon baking soda

- ¼ teaspoon salt

- 5 tablespoons unsalted butter, melted

- 2/3 cup (141 g) firmly packed light brown sugar

- 2/3 cup (131 g) sugar

- ¼ cup (60 ml) unsulphured molasses; not blackstrap

- 1 teaspoons cinnamon

- ½ teaspoon ground ginger

- 1/8 teaspoon ground cloves

- 1/8 teaspoon freshly grated nutmeg

- 1 cup (220 g) pure, unsweetened canned pumpkin

- 2 large eggs, at room temperature

PREPARATION:

1. Position rack in middle of oven. Preheat oven to 350°F (180°C). Coat the inside of a 9-inch (23 cspringform pan with nonstick spray; set aside.

2. For the Streusel: Mash together all of the streusel ingredients, except the pecans, in a small bowl. I like to start with a fork and then get in their with my fingers. The mixture should feel like wet sand, then mix in the chopped pecans; set aside.

3. For the Coffee Cake: Whisk together the flour, baking powder, baking soda and salt in a large mixing bowl to aerate and combine; set aside, making a well in the center.

4. In a separate bowl, whisk together the melted butter, sugars and molasses until well blended. Whisk in the spices, the canned pumpkin and then the eggs one at a time until everything comes together.

5. Scrape the pumpkin mixture on top of the dry mixture and whisk together until blended well and combined. Scrape batter into prepared pan and level the top. Scatter streusel evenly over the top.

6. Bake for 30 minutes, then cover with aluminum foil to keep the cake from browning too quickly and bake for about 20 minutes more or until a toothpick tests clean when inserted in the center of the cake. Cool cake on rack for at least 10 minutes, then unmold from springform pan. Cake may be served warm or cool to room temperature. Cake may be wrapped in foil and stored at room temperatures for up to 2 days.

Tips

- If you do not have a 9-inch (23 cm) round springform pan, make this cake in a 9-inch (23 cm) square pan. Cool completely. Do not unmold. Simply cut squares of the cake directly in the pan and lift out with a spatula.

Course: Breakfast, brunch, Snack

Cuisine: American

NUTRITION

Calories: 272kcal | Carbohydrates: 51g | Protein: 2g | Fat: 7g | Saturated Fat: 1g | Sodium: 141mg | Potassium: 62mg | Fiber: 1g | Sugar: 32g | Calcium: 12mg | Iron: 1mg

LEMONY LOW FODMAP CARBONARA

Our Lemony Low FODMAP Carbonara will curb any carb cravings you are having!

Makes: 6 Servings

Prep Time: 10 minutes

Cook Time: 20 minutes

Total Time: 30 minutes

INGREDIENTS:

- 16- ounces (455 g) low FODMAP gluten-free spaghetti, such as Jovial

- 1/4 cup (60 ml) extra virgin olive oil

- 6- ounces (170 g) guanciale, cut into 1/2 inch (12 mpieces

- 4 large egg yolks, at room temperature

- 1 1/2 cups (150 g) grated Parmigiano Reggiano, divided

- 2 tablespoons freshly squeezed lemon juice

- Lots of freshly cracked black pepper

- 1 teaspoon fine lemon zest

PREPARATION:

1. Bring a large pot of well salted water to a boil and cook pasta until it is just shy of "al dente" and still has a slight firmness, reserving 1 1/2 cups (360 ml) of starchy cooking liquid.

2. Meanwhile, heat olive oil in a 10 to 12 inch (25 cm to 30.5 cm) skillet over medium heat, add guanciale, and cook, stirring occasionally, until the pork fat begins to render and the guanciale lightly browns, about 5 minutes. Take off heat but keep warm.

3. While pasta is boiling and guanciale is cooking, break egg yolks into a large mixing bowl, stir in about 1 1/4 cups (125 g) of the cheese (mixture will look thick), stir in lemon juice and grind a generous amount of black pepper on top.

4. Once pasta is drained (with the 1 1/2 cups/360 ml of cooking water reserved), place skillet with guanciale back over very low heat, add pasta and quickly toss the pasta to coat for about 15 to 30 seconds; make sure the pasta is coated and warmed. REMOVE from heat.

5. Immediately add about 1/4 cup (60 ml) of the pasta water to your egg/cheese mixture and whisk to loosen. Quickly add this mixture to pasta and begin to toss. Add more pepper and water as you toss and a creamy sauce will develop (see Tips). Keep adding water and tossing until the pasta is coated with a rich, creamy sauce. Serve

immediately with more black pepper, reserved cheese and lemon zest on top.

Tips

• I love to make this dish with a combo of Parmigiano Reggiano and Pecorino Romano cheese. The extra-sharpness of the sheep milk based Romano adds another layer of flavor. Not necessary, but a great variation.

• The one tricky part of this dish is to not curdle the egg yolks. My technique recommends combining the ingredients off of the heat, so this should not happen. There is a stage during which you are tossing the pasta where you might think the mixture has curdled, but it is most likely that you just haven't added enough pasta water, which is integral to creating this "sauce". If your mixture looks sticky or gloppy, simply keep adding the reserved pasta water a little bit at a time. Toss as you go, until the mixture is silky and creamy. The pasta should look like it is coated with heavy cream and the reason why this dish is often mistakenly believed to contain cream.

- This delicious dish is rich in fat and should be enjoyed as a special occasion meal; tolerance to fat is very individual and can contribute to GI distress for some folks. Watch your portions; fill half your plate with a big green salad.

If You Can Tolerate

- Fructans: If you have passed the wheat fructan challenge feel free to use traditional pasta.

Course: Dinner, lunch, Main Course

Cuisine: Italian

NUTRITION

Calories: 700kcal | Carbohydrates: 57g | Protein: 21g | Fat: 44g | Saturated Fat: 9g | Cholesterol: 30mg | Sodium: 625mg | Fiber: 3g | Sugar: 1g | Iron: 1mg

MATZO BALL SOUP

Our Matzo Ball Soup uses low FODMAP gluten-free matzo, which may or may not be considered appropriate for your seder table. Please consult your rabbi. We think we have come up with a really great version. Enjoy!

Makes: 12 Servings

Prep Time: 15 minutes

Cook Time: 25 minutes

Total Time: 2 hours 40 minutes

INGREDIENTS:

Matzo Balls:

- 3 large eggs

- 3/4 cup (75 g) very finely ground low FODMAP gluten-free matzo meal

- 1/4 cup (60 ml) melted schmaltz (chicken fat) or vegetable oil

- 3 tablespoons club soda

- 1 teaspoon kosher salt

Soup:

- 24 cups (5.7 L) low FODMAP Chicken Stock, ready to use

- 2 medium carrots, peeled and cut into very thin (1/8-inch/3 mm) rounds

- 2 medium parsnips, peeled and cut into very thin (1/8-inch/3 mm) rounds

- Fresh dill

PREPARATION:

1. About 2 hours before serving, make the Matzo Ball mixture: whisk the eggs very well in a medium sized mixing bowl. Add the matzo meal, schmaltz, club soda and salt and stir together very well. The mixture will look wet. Cover with plastic wrap and refrigerate for 2 hours.

2. Bring a large pot of salted water to a boil. Meanwhile, use a small scoop to make approximately 2 tablespoon sized portions and use very wet hands to roll them into beautiful little balls. I roll the matzo balls one by one and lower them into the water as I go. Simmer the matzo balls for about 20 minutes. They should swell up and firm

up. Some recipes will tell you to cook until they sink; these will not sink.

3. Meanwhile, bring stock to a simmer and add your carrot and parsnip rounds and simmer for a few minutes until the vegetables are tender. Ladle soup and vegetables into individual soup dishes, add a matzo ball to each serving and garnish with fresh dill. Serve immediately.

Tips

- Sourcing the matzo might take some doing. I have had to resort to ordering on-line most of the time, so plan ahead.

Course: Appetizer, Soup

Cuisine: Jewish

NUTRITION

Calories: 265kcal | Carbohydrates: 24g | Protein: 14g | Fat: 12g | Saturated Fat: 1g | Cholesterol: 53mg | Sodium: 217mg | Potassium: 116mg | Fiber: 2g | Sugar: 8g | Vitamin A: 75IU | Vitamin C: 4.4mg | Calcium: 17mg | Iron: 0.4mg

FODMAP CUCUMBER GAZPACHO

This FODMAP Cucumber Gazpacho is very easy to make, but it does require and overnight sit in the refrigerator, so plan accordingly.

Low FODMAP Serving Size Info: Makes about 7 cups (1.7 L); serving size about 2 cups (480 ml)

Makes: 4 servings

Prep Time: 10 minutes

Chill Time 8 hours

Total Time: 8 hours 10 minutes

INGREDIENTS:

- 3 small (about 12 ounces (340 g) total) Persian cucumbers, (6-inch/15 cm each), ends trimmed away, cut into chunks, peel intact

- 2 large slices of sourdough bread about 1-inch (2.5 cm) thick and 8-inches (20 cm) across, torn into pieces

- 1/3 cups (50 g) toasted whole almonds, blanched or natural

- 4 cups (960 ml) unsweetened almond milk, such as Almond Breeze

- 2 tablespoons extra virgin olive oil or Garlic-Infused Oil, made with olive oil

- 2 tablespoons white wine vinegar

- 1 1/2 ounces (40 g) baby spinach

- 1/4 ounce (7 g) fresh mint leaves

- Kosher salt

- Freshly ground black pepper

PREPARATION:

1. Place cucumbers, bread and almonds in a large bowl (or blender carafe). Add the milk, oil and vinegar, cover, and refrigerate overnight.

2. Right before serving, scrape the mixture into your blender carafe (if it isn't in it already) and blend until very smooth. Add spinach and mint, blend again until smooth, then taste and season with salt and pepper as desired. Serve immediately.

Tips

- We always keep unsweetened almond milk in our Test Kitchen fridge. It is our go-to alt milk for cooking, especially savory. Try different brands to find one that you like.

Course: Appetizer, Soup

Cuisine: American

NUTRITION

Calories: 210kcal | Carbohydrates: 17g | Protein: 5g | Fat: 11g | Saturated Fat: 1g | Sodium: 10mg | Potassium: 69mg | Fiber: 1g | Sugar: 1g | Vitamin A: 1070IU | Vitamin C: 3.5mg | Calcium: 15mg | Iron: 0.4mg

LOW FODMAP SPICY SMOKY PUMPKIN SOUP

This low FODMAP soup is smooth, creamy and a little bit spicy! You CAN have pumpkin on the low FODMAP diet!

Low FODMAP Serving Size Info: Makes about 6 cups (1.4 L); serving size 1 cup (240 ml)

Makes: 6 servings

Prep Time: 10 minutes

Cook Time: 15 minutes

Total Time: 25 minutes

INGREDIENTS:

Soup:

- 2 tablespoons unsalted butter, cut into pieces

- 1 tablespoon Garlic-Infused Oil, made with olive oil, or purchased equivalent

- 3/4 cup chopped scallions, green parts only

- 1/2 teaspoon smoked paprika

- 1/4 teaspoon cinnamon

- 1/4 teaspoon nutmeg

- 1/8 teaspoon cayenne or to taste

- 3 cups (720 ml) water

- 2 teaspoons Fody Chicken Soup Base or Vegetable Soup Base

- 1, 15- ounce (425 g) can pure pumpkin, such as Libby's

- 1 tablespoon firmly packed light brown sugar

- 1 teaspoon kosher salt

- 3/4 cup (180 ml) lactose-free half and half, optional, and more as needed

- Freshly ground black pepper

Optional Toppings:

- Lactose-free sour cream, optional

- Toasted Pepitas, optional

PREPARATION:

1. Heat medium sized pot over low-medium heat, add butter and oil and cook until melted. Add scallions and

sauté a few minutes, stirring often until soft. Add smoked paprika, cinnamon, nutmeg, and 1/8 teaspoon cayenne and cook 15 seconds more.

2. Add water and soup base and whisk together well. Then whisk in canned pumpkin, brown sugar and salt. Bring to a simmer and cook for about 10 minutes, whisking occasionally. Cool slightly, add half and half, if using and then purée in blender until super smooth. Taste, add pepper and adjust salt, if desired. Soup is ready to serve; reheat if needed. You can thin it down a little more, if you like, with water, more half-and half or chicken or vegetable stock. If you want to make it a bit fancy, stir together a little lactose-free sour cream and drizzle on top an/or sprinkle on a few toasted pepitas. Soup can also be cooled and then refrigerated in an airtight container for up to 4 days.

Tip

- If you have an immersion blender, you could purée the soup right in the pot. Take care either way you blend it for splashes!

Course: Appetizer, Soup

Cuisine: American

NUTRITION

Calories: 143kcal | Carbohydrates: 9g | Protein: 3g | Fat: 11g | Saturated Fat: 1g | Sodium: 394mg | Fiber: 2g | Sugar: 4g | Vitamin A: 80IU | Calcium: 4mg

LOW FODMAP VEGETABLE, PASTA & BEAN SOUP

This Low FODMAP Vegetable, Pasta & Bean Soup is hearty and nourishing and happens to be vegan! Easy to make, too.

Low FODMAP Serving Size Info: Makes about 14 cups (3.3 L); about 10 servings; about 3/4 cup (180 ml) per serving.

Makes: 14 servings

Prep Time: 15 minutes

Cook Time: 30 minutes

Total Time: 45 minutes

INGREDIENTS:

- 2 tablespoons Garlic-Infused Oil, made with olive oil, or purchased equivalent

- 3/4 cup (48 g) finely chopped scallions, green parts only

- 1/4 cup (18 g) finely chopped leeks, green parts only

- 8 cups (2 L) water

- 1, 28- ounce (794 g) can crushed tomatoes

- 1, 15.5- ounce (439 g) can chickpeas, drained, rinsed and drained again

- 12- ounces (340 g) diced butternut squash

- 8- ounces (225 g) red potatoes, scrubbed and cut into small bite-sized pieces

- 6- ounces (170 g) cleaned and trimmed kale, chopped finely

- 3 medium carrots, scrubbed, trimmed and cut into thick rounds (1/2-inch/12 mm or even larger)

- 2 cups (150 g) sliced bok choy

- 1 medium yellow squash scrubbed, trimmed and cut into thick rounds (about 1/2-inch/12 mm thick)

- 1 medium zucchini scrubbed, trimmed, quartered and cut into small bite-sized pieces

- 1 teaspoon dried basil

- 1 teaspoon smoked paprika

- 1 teaspoon dried thyme

- Kosher salt

- Freshly ground black pepper

- 1 cup (100 g) raw gluten-free elbow or small shell shaped pasta

PREPARATION:

1. Place Garlic-Infused Oil in a large heavy pot or Dutch oven and heat over medium heat. Add scallion and leek greens and sauté for a few minutes until soft. Add water, canned tomatoes, chickpeas, squash, potatoes, kale, carrots, bok choy, yellow squash, zucchini, basil, smoked paprika and thyme and stir all together well. Season with salt and pepper.

2. Cover and bring to a boil over medium-high heat, then turn heat down and simmer for at least 30 minutes or until vegetables are tender, stirring occasionally. Taste and adjust seasoning as desired.

3. Meanwhile, cook pasta in a generous amount of salted water till al dente; drain and stir into soup (see Tips). Soup is ready to serve, or cool to room temperature and

refrigerate in an airtight container for up to 5 days. Reheat as needed.

Tips

• You could cook the pasta right in the soup, but it gives you bit less control over the pasta texture and the pasta also soaks up some of the luscious soup liquid, but if you are short on time or don't want to clean an extra pot, be our guest!

Course: Dinner, lunch, Soup

Cuisine: American & Italian

NUTRITION

Calories: 142kcal | Carbohydrates: 31g | Protein: 5g | Fat: 3g | Saturated Fat: 1g | Sodium: 7mg | Potassium: 3mg | Fiber: 3g | Sugar: 2g | Vitamin A: 70IU | Calcium: 7mg | Iron: 0.2mg

LOW FODMAP BOUILLABAISSE

Is Low FODMAP Bouillabaisse possible? Absolutely! We show you how to infuse garlic flavor without triggering your IBS!

Makes: 6 Servings

Prep Time: 15 minutes

Cook Time: 45 minutes

Total Time: 1 hour

INGREDIENTS:

Roasted Red Pepper Aioli:

- 1 large pasteurized egg yolk, at room temperature

- 2 teaspoons freshly squeezed lemon juice

- 1 teaspoon cold water

- ¼ teaspoon Dijon mustard

- Kosher salt

- 1 cup (240 ml) Garlic-Infused Oil, made with olive oil, or purchased equivalent

- ½ cup (85 g) very finely chopped, drained jarred roasted red peppers

- Cayenne pepper

- Freshly ground black pepper

Toast:

- 1, low FODMAP French baguette

- 2 tablespoons Garlic-Infused Oil, made with olive oil, or equivalent

Bouillabaisse:

- ¾ pound (340 g) large (26 to 30 count) shrimp, deveined, shells on

- ¼ cup (60 ml) Garlic-Infused Oil, made with olive oil, or purchased equivalent

- 1 cup (140 g) finely chopped leeks, green parts only

- 1 cup (98 g) thinly sliced fresh fennel bulb; reserve some fennel fronds (the delicate, feathery tops)

- 3 canned plum tomatoes, drained of juice, chopped

- 2 tablespoons chopped fresh flat-leaf parsley

- 2 teaspoons finely grated orange zest

- 1 teaspoon chopped fresh thyme

- ½ teaspoon fennel seeds, crushed

- 24 small or medium-size clams or mussels or preferably a combination of both, scrubbed free of sand and grit; de-beard the mussels if necessary

- 1½ pounds (680 g) white flesh fish, preferably more than one kind, such as cod fillets, cod loins, red snapper, halibut, haddock, monkfish, or striped bass, cut into chunks

- ¾ pound (340 g) sea scallops; cut in half if very large

- 1 tablespoon chopped fresh basil

- Kosher salt

- Freshly ground black pepper

PREPARATION:

1. For the Aioli: Place the pasteurized egg yolk, lemon juice, cold water, mustard, and ½ teaspoon of salt in a

medium-size nonreactive bowl. Whisk vigorously until blended. Very slowly, drop by drop, whisk in about a quarter of the olive oil, whisking all the while. This will take several minutes; go slowly, allowing the mayonnaise to thicken. Gradually add the remaining olive oil until the desired thickness is reached; you might not use all the oil, but you will most likely use at least ¾ cup (180 ml). Gently stir in the chopped peppers and cayenne to taste.

2. Season to taste with more salt and with black pepper, if desired. The aioli is ready to use, or refrigerate in an airtight container for up to 2 days.

3. For the Toast: Right before beginning to cook the seafood, slice the baguette into 1-inch (2.5 cm) slices, toast in a toaster or on a baking sheet in a 400°F (200°C) oven, then brush with the olive oil; set aside.

4. For the Bouillabaisse: Peel the shrimp and set them aside, reserving shells. Place the shells in a medium-size saucepan with 4½ cups (1 L) of water. Bring to a boil, lower the heat, and simmer for 5 minutes. This is a super-quick shellfish stock.

5. While the shrimp shells are simmering, heat the oil in a deep 5-quart (4.7 L) pot, such as a Dutch oven, over medium heat. Add the leek greens and sliced fennel and sauté for 3 to 5 minutes, or until softened but not browned.

6. Strain and measure out 4 cups (960 ml) of the stock for the bouillabaisse. Discard the shells. Add the shrimp stock, tomatoes, parsley, orange zest, thyme, and fennel seeds to the leek mixture. Cover, increase the heat, and simmer for 10 minutes

7. Add the clams and/or mussels, cover, and cook for about 5 minutes, or until the shells open, discarding any that do not open. Add the white fish and scallops, cover, and cook for about 5 minutes, or until the fish is almost opaque. Add the shrimp and cook, covered, for about 3 to 5 minutes more, or just until the shrimp turn pink. Gently stir in the basil and taste the broth. Season with salt and pepper, as desired.

8. Place a slice or two of garlic toast in each bowl and top the toasts with a generous dollop of aioli. Ladle the stew on top and garnish with fennel fronds, if you like. Serve immediately.

Tips

- If you want to make a Roasted Red Pepper Aioli using prepared mayo, you can, but you will be missing out on the potent garlic flavor. Simply stir together ½ cup (113 g) of prepared mayonnaise, ¼ cup (85 g) of drained and chopped jarred roasted red peppers, 2 teaspoons of freshly squeezed lemon juice, and ⅛ teaspoon cayenne pepper in a food processor and pulse one and off just until combined. Season to taste with salt and black pepper; the quickie aioli is ready to use.

Course: Dinner

Cuisine: American, French

NUTRITION

Calories: 1116kcal | Carbohydrates: 20g | Protein: 78g | Fat: 70g | Sodium: 123mg | Fiber: 1g | Sugar: 2g | Calcium: 30mg

LOW FODMAP GAZPACHO

Our Low FODMAP Gazpacho has garlic and onion favor, but won't upset your tummy!

Low FODMAP Serving Size Info: Makes about 4 cups (960 ml); 4, (1 cup/240 ml) servings

Makes: 4 Servings

Prep Time: 15 minutes

Cook Time: 5 minutes

Total Time: 20 minutes

INGREDIENTS:

- 2- pounds (910 g) fresh super-ripe red tomatoes, peeled, seeded, cored and very finely chopped

- 1 cup (70 g) very finely chopped scallions, green parts only

- Half a hothouse English cucumber, about 6-inches (15 cm), peeled, seeded and very finely chopped

- ½ green bell pepper, cored, very finely chopped

- ½ red bell pepper, cored, very finely chopped

- 2 tablespoons Garlic-Infused Oil, made with olive oil, or purchased equivalent, plus extra

- 1 to 2 tablespoons red wine vinegar, or sherry vinegar

- Kosher salt

- Freshly ground black pepper

- Tabasco; optional

- Fresh herbs; optional, such as marjoram or basil

- Hunk of sourdough bread, equivalent to a large slice, torn into bite-sized pieces

PREPARATION:

1. Stir together your chopped tomatoes, with any juice, with the scallions, cucumber and bell peppers in a nonreactive bowl. Stir in 1 tablespoon of the garlic-infused olive oil. Add about a quarter of the soup mixture to your blender carafe and purée, then stir the purée back into the main mixture.

2. Taste and add vinegar to taste along with salt and pepper. Add Tabasco if you like. The soup is ready to serve but I think it is even better after it has sit for about 1 hour for flavors to meld. You can also refrigerate it in an airtight container for up to 1 day, but the brightness of the vegetable flavors will mute.

3. For the croutons, heat some of the extra Garlic-Infused Oil in a nonstick pan over medium-high heat, add the sourdough bread chunks and sprinkle with some salt. Toss to coat with oil and cook until toasted and golden

brown, tossing several times during cooking for even browning; set aside.

4. Serve the gazpacho in bowls, or small glasses for sipping. A larger glass for an appetizer, or a tiny glass for a passed hors d'oeuvres is fantastic.

5. Drizzle with remaining 1 tablespoon Garlic-Infused Oil right before serving and add fresh herbs if you like. Top with crunchy croutons and serve. SUMMER IN A BOWL!

Tips

- To Peel Tomatoes: Bring a large pot of water to a boil. Drop whole tomatoes into the water and blanch for about a minute or until the skin slips off easily. Carefully remove from water and drain. Allow to cool until you can handle them comfortably. Slip off the peels and discard. Slice in half crosswise and squeeze out and discard the seeds. I use my fingers to help. Your tomatoes are now ready to chop. Chop them on a cutting board that will catch all the juice and add that to your recipe as well.

Course: Appetizer, Dinner & Lunch, Soup

Cuisine: Spanish

NUTRITION

Calories: 125kcal | Carbohydrates: 18g | Protein: 4g | Fat: 7g | Sodium: 1mg | Fiber: 2g | Sugar: 4g

LOW FODMAP VEGETABLE BROTH

Low FODMAP Vegetable Broth couldn't be easier. Just give yourself time for it to simmer on the stove.

Low FODMAP Serving Size Info: Makes about 4 quarts (3.8 L); serving size up to 1 cup (240 ml); 8 servings

Makes: 8 servings

Prep Time: 15 minutes

Cook Time: 1 hour

Total Time: 1 hour 15 minutes

INGREDIENTS:

- 2 tablespoons Low FODMAP Garlic-Infused Oil made with olive oil or vegetable oil, or purchased equivalent such as FODY Garlic-Infused Olive Oil

- 1 cup (72 g) chopped leeks, green parts only, divided

- 1 cup (64 g) chopped scallions, green parts only, divided

- 1 large bunch fresh flat leaf parsley roughly chopped

- 6 medium sprigs of fresh thyme

- 1 teaspoon black peppercorns

- 1 large bay leaf

- 3 medium carrots, scrubbed, peel intact, cut into 1-inch (24 mm) pieces

- 2 medium gold or white potatoes, scrubbed and quartered

- 2 medium parsnips, 225 g, scrubbed, ends trimmed and sliced into 1/2-inch (12 mm) rounds

- 1 medium fennel bulb, root end trimmed away, bulb sliced and fronds (the top, feathery leaves) and stems chopped

- 1 medium celery stalk, cut into 1-inch (24 mm) pieces

- 1 tablespoon kosher salt

- Water

PREPARATION:

1. Add the oil to a 5 to 6 quart (4.7 L to 5.7 L) stockpot and heat over low-medium heat. Add half of the leek and scallion greens (just eyeball it) and sauté, stirring frequently, for a few minutes until softened. Add parsley, thyme, peppercorns, bay leaf, carrots, remaining leek and scallion greens, potatoes, parsnips, fennel, celery and salt to the pot.

2. Add enough cold water to cover the vegetables by about 2-inches (5 cm). Cover pot and bring to a simmer over medium heat; adjust heat and cook at a gentle simmer for 1 hour. Skim off any froth that rises to the top during the first half hour. Check occasionally and add water if necessary to keep all solid ingredients just submerged. Taste for flavor. If the broth seems weak, keep simmering for a while. You might also want to adjust salt level.

3. Strain into a clean pot or storage container(s) and discard solids. Allow broth to cool to room temperature, then refrigerate overnight. Skim all of the fat off of the surface, if desired. Divide the broth into airtight containers in small portions for ease of use. We like to make 1 cup (240 ml) and 2 cup (480 ml) amounts in particular and either refrigerate up to a 3 days or freeze

for up to 6 months. You can also freeze the broth in ice cube trays, then pop out the cubes once frozen and freeze in heavy plastic zipper top bags.

Tips

- If you are not vegan and want to try an extra ingredient that adds tons of flavor, add a big hunk of parmesan cheese rind with the rest of the ingredients during simmering. It adds flavor as well as a little body.

If You Can Tolerate Fructans:

- If you have passed the Onion Fructan Challenge, feel free to use a white or yellow onion or two (to your tolerance) in lieu of the leeks and scallions, and it may be left in during simmering.

- If you have passed the Garlic Fructan Challenge, feel free to use minced garlic (to your tolerance), added at the beginning and sautéed, and it may be left in during simmering.

Polyols:

- If you have passed the mannitol Challenge consider adding up to 3 stalks of celery. It adds such a wonderful flavor to soup bases.

Course: Basic, Soup

Cuisine: American

NUTRITION

Calories: 113kcal | Carbohydrates: 17g | Protein: 2g | Fat: 4g | Saturated Fat: 1g | Sodium: 872mg | Potassium: 7mg | Fiber: 2g | Sugar: 3g | Calcium: 2mg | Iron: 0.1mg

LOW FODMAP CLAM CHOWDER

This is a New England style Low FODMAP Clam Chowder to satisfy your soup yearnings!

Low FODMAP Serving Size Info: Makes about 10 cups (2.4 L); serves 8

Makes: 8 Servings

Prep Time: 20 minutes

Cook Time: 20 minutes

Total Time: 40 minutes

INGREDIENTS:

Broth:

- 8- pounds (3.6 kg) cherrystone or quahog clams (see Tips

- 2 cups (480 ml) water

Chowder:

- 4- ounces (115 g) thick-cut bacon chopped into small pieces

- 3 tablespoons unsalted butter

- 1 tablespoon Garlic-Infused Oil, made with vegetable oil, or purchased equivalent

- 3/4 cup (54 g) finely chopped leeks, green parts only

- 3/4 cup (48 g) finely chopped scallions, green parts only

- 1 stalk celery, trimmed and diced

- 2 teaspoons fresh thyme leaves

- 2- pounds (910 g) russet baking potatoes peeled and cut into large bite-sized chunks

- 1 large bay leaf

- 2 cups (480 ml) lactose free heavy cream, at room temperature

- Freshly ground black pepper

- Finely chopped fresh flat leaf parsley

- Snipped fresh chives

PREPARATION:

1. For the Broth: Scrub the clams well to remove any grit with cool water. Place clams in a very large stockpot along with the 2 cups (480 mof water. Cover and bring to a low boil over medium heat; after 5 minutes stir the clams with a sturdy wooden spoon to get the ones on top down to the bottom and vice versa. Cover and cook for about 5 minutes more or just until clams open. Timing will vary depending on size of clams; some will open fully while others will only open a tiny bit, which is fine.

Remove from heat. If any clams remain shut tight, discard them.

2. Use tongs to pick the clams up one by one, tipping any captured broth in the shells back into the pot. Place clamshells with clams in strainer. Some clams will have fallen out of their shells into the broth, which is okay. Pick clams out of shells in strainer and place on a cutting board and use tongs to remove any loose clams from broth and place them on cutting board, too. Discard shells. The clams can cool briefly before chopping, while you strain the broth.

3. Set a wire-mesh strainer lined with a double-layer of cheesecloth over a large measuring cup. Pour broth through cheesecloth; there might be some grit, which you will capture and leave behind. (The grit will be on the bottom of your cup and you can also stop short of

pouring out that last grit-filled bit for extra insurance). Set broth aside momentarily.

4. Chop the clams on the cutting board and refrigerate until needed.

5. For the Chowder: Wipe out the original stockpot and add bacon. Cook over low-medium heat to render the fat and cook until bacon is crisp. Remove bacon bits and reserve, draining on paper towels. Add butter and oil, chopped leeks, scallions, celery and thyme and sauté gently over low-medium heat for about 5 minutes or until vegetables are soft but not browned.

6. Taste the strained broth. If it is very strong it will have a very briny, salty flavor, in which case I suggest using part water and not all of the broth. You have to use your taste buds here. Remember that you will be adding

cream later, so that flavor will be tempered regardless, but if it is very strong you will know it!

7. You need a total of 4-cups (960 mof liquid, either all broth or part broth and part water. Add the 4-cups (960 mliquid to the pot along with the potatoes and bay leaf. Cover the pot and bring to a low boil over medium-high heat and cook until potatoes are soft, about 10 to 15 minutes. Use the back of a wooden spoon or a potato masher to mash some of the potatoes right in the pot. Their starch will add richness to the chowder.

8. Add the reserved bacon, chopped clams and the cream and heat over low heat until very hot, but do not boil. Taste and add pepper as desired. Soup is ready to serve but improves after it sits for an hour. Serve with parsley and chives sprinkled on top. The un-garnished chowder can be refrigerated overnight and reheated very gently

without simmering or boiling; the flavors (particularly the saltiness and clam essencmight intensify, which you can address by adding more water or cream.

Tips

• The size clams that you can find might vary and you might come across terms like "littleneck", "cherrystone" and "quahog" or "chowder" clams. They are all versions of hard-shelled clams and can be used for this chowder; just go by weight when purchasing. We prefer using cherrystones or the larger quahogs/chowder clams; just don't mix them in your stockpot as they will steam open at different rates.

Course: Appetizer, Dinner & Lunch, Soup

Cuisine: American

NUTRITION

Calories: 456kcal | Carbohydrates: 27g | Protein: 14g | Fat: 26g | Saturated Fat: 2g | Cholesterol: 9mg | Sodium: 97mg | Potassium: 28mg | Fiber: 2g | Sugar: 1g | Vitamin A: 24IU | Vitamin C: 1mg | Calcium: 4mg | Iron: 1mg

LOW FODMAP OYSTER MUSHROOM GRAVY

Low FODMAP Oyster Mushroom Gravy is easy to make and takes advantage of oyster mushrooms, which are low FODMAP in 1 cup (75 g) amounts.

Low FODMAP Serving Size Info: Makes about 4 to 5 cups (960 ml to 1.2 L); serving size 2 tablespoons

Makes: 40 servings

Prep Time: 10 minutes

Cook Time: 10 minutes

Total Time: 20 minutes

INGREDIENTS:

- 1/2 cup (1 stick; 113 g) unsalted butter, cut into pieces

- 1/2 cup (40 g) finely chopped scallions, green parts only

- 5- ounces (140 g) trimmed and cleaned oyster mushrooms, chopped

- 1/2 cup (73 g) low FODMAP, gluten-free all-purpose flour

- 5 cups (1.2) warm low FODMAP chicken or turkey stock; make it conveniently with Fody Chicken Soup Base

- Kosher salt

- Freshly cracked black pepper

- Pan drippings, optional but highly recommended

PREPARATION:

1. Melt the butter in a medium sized saucepan over low-medium heat. Add scallions and mushrooms and sauté, stirring often, until the vegetables are softened, about 4 to 5 minutes.

2. Sprinkle flour over vegetable mixture and whisk in to blend. Turn heat up to medium and cook for a minute or two or until flour just begins to color.

3. Slowly add about 4 cups (960 ml) of stock, whisking all the while, until smooth. Continue to cook, whisking occasionally, until gravy begins to thicken. This will only take a few minutes. Add additional stock if necessary to achieve a nice thick but flowable gravy. Whisk until smooth. Season to taste with salt and pepper taking into consideration that you will need less (especially salt) if you will be adding pan drippings. We do think that a generous amount of pepper improves the gravy greatly.

4. The gravy is ready to use, or you may whisk in pan drippings at this time, in which case the color will be greatly enriched. You may also cool the gravy at this point (before or after adding pan drippings) and then

refrigerate in an airtight container for up to 3 days. Reheat over low heat on the stovetop when needed

If You Can Tolerate

- If you have passed the fructan wheat Challenge, and do not need to eat gluten-free, you can use regular wheat based all-purpose flour.

Course: Condiment

Cuisine: American

NUTRITION

Calories: 43kcal | Carbohydrates: 4g | Protein: 1g | Fat: 3g | Sodium: 110mg | Fiber: 1g | Sugar: 1g

LOW FODMAP SPOOKY GRAVEYARD 7-LAYER DIP

Our Low FODMAP Spooky Graveyard 7-Layer Dip has all the familiar flavors you crave - assembled a little differently to create an unforgettable seasonal treat.

Low FODMAP Serving Size Info: Makes LOTS of servings; serving size is approximately 2 tablespoons worth. Just take 2 chips, dig in and enjoy!

Makes: 24 servings at least

Prep Time: 15 minutes

Cook Time: 10 minutes

Total Time: 25 minutes

INGREDIENTS:

- 2, 8 to 10- inch (20 cm to 25 c) brown rice tortillas

- Nonstick spray

- Black edible black pen

- 3 cups (720 g) lactose-free sour cream

- 2 cups (100 g) very finely shredded iceberg lettuce

- 6 ounces (170 g) shredded cheddar (we used a blend of white and orange)

- 2 medium plum tomatoes, cored and diced

- 1/2 cup (60 g) sliced black olives

- 2 cups (480 ml) guacamole

- 2, 16- ounce (453 g each) jars low FODMAP salsa

- 1/4 cup (16 g) chopped scallions, green parts only

- Plastic Halloween toys as desired

PREPARATION:

1. Position rack in middle of oven. Preheat oven to 350°F/180°C.

2. Cut out the tree and tombstone shapes from the flour tortillas. I traced shapes with an edible pen first for the tree, to help. Lightly spray the pieces with nonstick spray and place on baking sheet pan. Bake for about 5 to 10 minutes or until lightly tinged with color. Cool completely on pan on rack. Use edible black pen to write whatever you like on the stones. Set aside.

3. If your salsa is very liquidy, set a wire-mesh strainer over a bowl and pour the salsa into the strainer to drain for about 5 minutes. You want some of the liquid to drain away.

4. Take your "graveyard" container of choice and assemble your ingredients: spread the sour cream evenly

all over the bottom, then scatter the lettuce on top and gently press down into the lactose free sour cream. Top with cheddar cheese then tomatoes and olives. Spread the guacamole all over the top; it should reach from edge to edge to create a base for the salsa. Gently spoon the salsa all over the top. The Low FODMAP Spooky Graveyard 7-Layer Dip can be held for a few hours at this point in the refrigerator; after about 4 hours it can become watery, so plan accordingly. Right before serving, sprinkle scallion greens here and there and place the tree and gravestones, gently pressing down into the "soil".

5. Serve with low FODMAP corn chips and wait for the oohs and aahs.

Tips

- We are dedicated to helping you THRIVE during the holidays! Simply search by Holiday name and find dozens and dozens of low FODMAP recipe.

Course: Side Dish, Snack

Cuisine: American

NUTRITION

Calories: 141kcal | Carbohydrates: 7g | Protein: 4g | Fat: 12g | Saturated Fat: 1g | Sodium: 170mg | Potassium: 96mg | Fiber: 2g | Sugar: 2g | Vitamin A: 30IU | Vitamin C: 2mg | Calcium: 2mg | Iron: 0.1mg

LOW FODMAP SWEET & SPICY DRY RUB

Our version of Low FODMAP Sweet & Spicy Dry Rub combines cumin with both sweet and smoked paprika as well as brown sugar and other spices. Use with any protein!

Low FODMAP Serving Size Info: This makes about 1/2 cup (about 40 g); serving size is hard to gauge as you will be rubbing it into various serving sizes of protein; start with 2 teaspoons of rub to assess tolerance.

Makes: 12 servings

Prep Time: 5 minutes

Total Time: 5 minutes

INGREDIENTS:

- 2 tablespoons firmly packed light brown sugar

- 2 tablespoons kosher salt

- 1 tablespoon smoked paprika

- 1 tablespoon sweet paprika

- 1 tablespoon ground cumin

- 1 tablespoon freshly ground black pepper

- 1 teaspoon chipotle chile powder, or to taste, or use cayenne

PREPARATION:

1. Combine all the dry rub ingredients in a mixing bowl, use your fingers to break up any lumps of brown sugar, and mix everything together.

2. When applying to your fish, meat or poultry I like to use my hands to really rub it in.

3. Use right away or store in an airtight container for up to 1 week.

Tips

- Make sure that your spices are fresh! Buy what you need and that you can use within 6 months and store in a cool, dark area in airtight containers.

Course: Basic, Condiment

Cuisine: American

NUTRITION

Calories: 15kcal | Carbohydrates: 3g | Protein: 1g | Fat: 1g | Saturated Fat: 1g | Sodium: 1164mg | Potassium: 36mg | Fiber: 1g | Sugar: 2g | Vitamin A: 580IU | Calcium: 7mg | Iron: 0.6mg

LOW FODMAP PINEAPPLE SALSA

This Low FODMAP Pineapple Salsa comes together in a flash, especially if you buy peeled and cored fresh pineapple.

Low FODMAP Serving Size Info: Makes 1 1/2 cups (240 g); serving size 2 tablespoons

Makes: 12 servings

Prep Time: 5 minutes

Total Time: 5 minutes

INGREDIENTS:

- 1 cup (6 ounces/170 g) diced pineapple

- 1/2 medium red bell pepper, cored and diced

- 3 tablespoons finely chopped scallions, green parts only

- 2 tablespoons finely chopped cilantro

- Minced jalapeno to taste

- Kosher salt

- Lime juice

PREPARATION:

1. Stir together the pineapple, red pepper, scallion and cilantro. Add jalapeno - start with 1 teaspoon. Taste and adjust jalapeno and add salt and lime juice to your preference. This is ALL about the balance between the heat (jalapeno), salt and acid (lime). Just tinker until you love it. This Low FODMAP Pineapple Salsa is ready to use but it does improve after a 30-minute rest for flavors to meld. It is best if used the day it is made. Refrigerate in an airtight container until needed if you won't be using it for several hours.

Tips

- We love buying our pineapple pre-cut. Price-wise it actually ends up being very reasonable because there is no waste. Saves time, too.

Course: Condiment

Cuisine: American

NUTRITION

Calories: 11kcal | Carbohydrates: 2g

LOW FODMAP RED WINE VINAIGRETTE

Our Low FODMAP Red Wine Vinaigrette takes less than 5 minutes to prepare and can enliven so many different salads.

Low FODMAP Serving Size Info: Makes about 1 cup (240 ml); serving size 2 tablespoons

Makes: 8 servings

Prep Time: 5 minutes

Total Time: 5 minutes

INGREDIENTS:

- 3/4 cup (180 ml) extra-virgin olive oil

- 1/3 cup (75 ml) red wine vinegar

- 1 tablespoon Dijon mustard, such as Grey Poupon

- Kosher salt, optional

- Freshly ground black pepper, optional

PREPARATION:

1. Shake the oil, vinegar and mustard together in a glass covered jar. Season with salt and pepper to taste, if desired, but highly recommended. The vinaigrette is ready to use or may be refrigerated in a covered container for up to a week. Bring to room temperature before using. You can warm the jar in a bowl of warm water if you are in a rush. Shake well right before using.

DÉDÉ'S QUICK RECIPE TIPS VIDEO

Tips

- We like a sharp vinaigrette with a slightly higher ratio of vinegar; the classic ratio is 3 to 1 oil to vinegar. We encourage you to use this recipe as a baseline but you can play with the ratios to your taste.

Course: Basic

Cuisine: American, French

NUTRITION

Calories: 199kcal | Carbohydrates: 1g | Protein: 1g | Fat: 22g | Saturated Fat: 3g | Sodium: 23mg | Fiber: 1g | Sugar: 1g | Iron: 0.2mg

LOW FODMAP MINT SALSA VERDE

Our Low FODMAP Mint Salsa Verde uses fresh parsley and mint with tangy anchovies to make a vibrant sauce that goes beautifully with low FODMAP main proteins.

Low FODMAP Serving Size: Makes about 1 cup (240 ml); serving size 2 tablespoons

Makes: 8 servings

Prep Time: 10 minutes

Total Time: 10 minutes

INGREDIENTS:

- 1/2 cup (120 ml) Garlic-Infused Oil, made with olive oil
- 3 tablespoons freshly squeezed lemon juice
- 1 cup (16 g) parsley leaves
- 1/2 cup (8 g) mint leaves

- 1/2 cup (32 g) chopped scallions, green parts only

- 2 flat oil-packed anchovy filets

- 1 tablespoon drained brine-packed capers

- Kosher salt

- Freshly ground black pepper

PREPARATION:

1. Place the olive oil and lemon juice in blender, then add parsley, mint, scallions, anchovies and capers. Pulse the blender on and off then blend until the sauce is smooth, scraping down the blender carafe as needed. Taste and season with salt and pepper. The Low FODMAP Mint Salsa Verde is ready to use or may be refrigerated overnight and brought back to room temperature before using. If it has separated, whisk it together vigorously before using.

Tips

- It is imperative to make this with FRESH herbs! Do not try this with dried.

Course: Sauce

Cuisine: American

Tags: Low FODMAP Recipes for the Fourth of July, Low FODMAP Summer Recipe Roundup

NUTRITION

Calories: 144kcal | Carbohydrates: 4g | Protein: 2g | Fat: 14g | Saturated Fat: 1g | Sodium: 58mg | Potassium: 248mg | Fiber: 2g | Sugar: 1g | Vitamin A: 3120IU | Vitamin C: 44.1mg | Calcium: 77mg | Iron: 2.6mg

LOW FODMAP MISO COD RAMEN

This Low FODMAP Miso Cod Ramen is from the book Wagamama Feed Your Soul, in which we found much inspiration.

Makes: 2 Servings

Prep Time: 10 minutes

Cook Time: 10 minutes

Marination Time: 30 minutes

Total Time: 50 minutes

INGREDIENTS:

Cod Marinade:

- 1 tablespoon white miso paste

- 2 teaspoons mirin

- 1 tablespoon soy sauce

- 1- inch (2.5 cm) piece of ginger, peeled and grated

- 1 tablespoon sesame oil

- 4 cod fillets, about 455 g, with skin, cut into 2 pieces

Vegetables & Soba:

- 3 tablespoons vegetable oil

- 6 1/2- ounces (180 g) cooked soba noodles, kept warm

- 2 cups (150 g) chopped bok choi

- 2¼ cups (540 ml) low FODMAP Vegetable Broth

- 2 teaspoons soy sauce

- 1 teaspoon oyster sauce

- 1 tablespoon fish sauce

Garnish:

- 2 scallions, green parts only, finely sliced

- 12 pieces bamboo shoots

- 1 tablespoon chili oil to taste

PREPARATION:

1. For the Cod Marinade: Place the marinade ingredients in a wide, shallow bowl and stir to combine. Add the cod fillets and coat well, then cover and leave to marinate in the fridge for at least 30 minutes.

2. Cook the Fish, Vegetables & Soba: Heat 2 tablespoons of the vegetable oil in a skillet or wok over medium heat until hot and place the cod fillets, skin-side down, into the pan. Pan-fry the fish for 2 to 3 minutes until the

skin is golden brown, then turn and cook for a further 2 to 3 minutes on the other side. Transfer the fish to a plate and set aside.

3. Add the remaining 1 tablespoon oil to the wok and stir-fry the bok choi until it starts to wilt. Add the vegetable stock to the wok with the soy, oyster, and fish sauces and stir to heat through.

4. Divide the cooked noodles between 2 serving bowls and add the broth. Top with the bok choi and cod and garnish with the scallions, menma, and a drizzle of chili oil, to taste.

Tips

- I love that this dish features traditional soba! The low FODMAP diet is not a gluten-free diet and soba noodles, in the amounts suggested here, are allowed - and encouraged!

Course: Appetizer, Dinner, lunch, Main Course, Soup

Cuisine: Asian

NUTRITION

Calories: 619kcal | Carbohydrates: 27g | Protein: 49g | Fat: 36g | Saturated Fat: 2g | Sodium: 1991mg | Potassium: 37mg | Fiber: 1g | Sugar: 3g | Iron: 1mg

LOW FODMAP BREAKFAST CASSEROLE

Our Low FODMAP Breakfast Casserole can be prepped the night before and is the perfect dish for holidays and brunches.

Makes: 14 Servings

Prep Time: 5 minutes

Cook Time: 1 hour

Total Time: 1 hour 5 minutes

INGREDIENTS:

- 24- ounce to 30-ounce (680 g to 685 g) package of low FODMAP frozen hash browns, about 8 to 9 cups

- 1- pound (455 g) thickly sliced low FODMAP ham, diced

- 8- ounces (225 g) sharp cheddar cheese, shredded

- 12 large eggs

- 1 cup (240 ml) lactose-free whole milk

- Kosher salt

- Freshly ground black pepper

PREPARATION:

1. Position rack in middle of oven. Preheat oven to 350°C (180°C). Coat the inside of a 13-inch by 9-inch (33 cm by 23 cm) casserole dish with nonstick spray; set aside.

2. Toss together the frozen hash browns, ham and cheese in a large bowl to evenly combine, then scrape into prepared pan, creating an even layer.

3. In same bowl, whisk the eggs and milk until thoroughly combined. Season with salt and pepper, then pour evenly over the potato mixture. Gently pat everything down with the back of a sturdy spoon.

4. Bake for one hour, uncovered or until the center is set and the edges are golden brown. Let sit for 5 minutes and serve.

Tips

- I like to serve low FODMAP hot sauce or salsa alongside. Some folks like ketchup with their eggs, and since there are low FODMAP serving sizes, why not offer it? We have a great article on Condiments, by the way.

Course: Breakfast, brunch

Cuisine: American

NUTRITION

Calories: 216kcal | Carbohydrates: 12g | Protein: 15g | Fat: 17g | Sodium: 151mg

Made in the USA
Monee, IL
04 June 2022

97489801R00073